Anchors for Bipolar Disorder

Building a Life of Stability with the Right Care Team, Community, and Rhythms

Dr. Cindy H. Carr, D.Min. MACL

The Anchored Series

Printed in the United States of America
First Edition, 2026

ISBN: 978-1-971192-22-2

For permissions or inquiries, contact:
Cindy H. Carr
cindyhcarr@outlook.com
www.cindyhcarr.com

Dedication

To the ones who have tried to hold it together while their brain changed the rules. And to the people who stayed—steadfast, educated, and kind.

Foreword

Some people know you long before they ever know your diagnosis, and that changes how they show up when life falls apart. Dr. Cindy H. Carr has known me since kindergarten, and when a legal crisis hit my life in 2013, she reached out because she could tell something was not right. She stayed close through my hospitalization and after. I am deeply grateful for the time, care, and work she invested in helping me understand bipolar disorder and build real stability. Her anchors framework became the foundation for what I now call my Four Pillars Model: psychiatry, therapy, family, and faith community, which I use in my own life and share with others through my coaching. Living with bipolar disorder is hard, but it does not have to define you. My hope is that this book helps you find your grounding and live anchored, too.

-Christopher Aldana

How to Use This Book

This book is designed to meet you in real life—not only in your best moments.

If you're stable right now: read straight through. Highlight what sounds like you. Complete the planning tools slowly, ideally with your psychiatrist, therapist, and a trusted support person.

If you're not stable right now: start with the shortest, most stabilizing chapters first—especially Sleep and Daily Rhythms and Planning for Escalation. Keep your reading simple and practical.

If you're newly diagnosed: take this one anchor at a time. Your first win is not "never having symptoms." Your first win is building a foundation strong enough to catch things early.

If you've been living with bipolar for years: you're not behind. You're here. We'll focus on reducing the cost of episodes and increasing your ability to return to your values sooner.

What to keep in mind as you read: When bipolar symptoms rise, your brain can become less reliable at judging risk, consequence, and urgency. That is why so many tools in this book are about planning while you are well—so your stable self can protect your future self.

A Note to the Reader

This book is educational and supportive. It is not a substitute for medical care, psychiatric evaluation, psychotherapy, diagnosis, or individualized treatment planning. Depression is a serious medical condition. The safest foundation for long-term stability is ongoing care with qualified professionals—especially a therapist and, when appropriate, a psychiatrist or other psychiatric prescriber.

If you are in immediate danger, thinking about harming yourself or someone else, unable to keep yourself safe, or experiencing severe impairment, seek urgent help right away. In the United States, you can call or text 988 (the Suicide & Crisis Lifeline). If you are outside the U.S., contact your local emergency number or crisis service.

Nothing in this book should be used to delay emergency care. If you are unsure, choose safety and reach out now.

Language note: This book uses practical terms like "yellow zone" and "red zone" to describe early warning signs and escalation. These terms are not clinical diagnoses; they are tools to help you respond earlier and reduce harm in real life.

Table of Contents

Introduction
This Is a Serious Medical Condition—and You Can Build a Stable Life

The Anchors framework emerged from years of pastoral counseling practice and was shaped through doctoral-level work focused on collaborative care for mental illness. Earlier versions of these ideas—then described as "pillars"—were developed, implemented, and evaluated within supervised ministry settings alongside licensed clinicians, caregivers, and individuals living with serious mental illness. The current Anchors model represents a refined, simplified adaptation designed specifically for people living with mental illness.

If you are holding this book in your hands, you may have lived through seasons where your brain seemed to change the rules without warning—where sleep became slippery, emotions ran too high or too low, and decisions felt urgent, obvious, or impossible. You may have tried to white-knuckle your way through it. You may have been told to "try harder," "calm down," or "be more disciplined." And you may have discovered, the hard way, that bipolar disorder does not respond well to shame or willpower alone.

Let me say this clearly from the beginning: bipolar disorder is a serious medical condition. It is a brain health issue that affects mood regulation, energy, motivation, sleep, and the speed and intensity of thought. It can be disruptive. It can be dangerous. And it deserves real care.

It is also treatable. Many people with bipolar disorder learn to reduce the frequency, severity, and cost of episodes. They build routines that protect stability. They strengthen relationships and repair what has been broken. They learn how to ask for help early— before a spiral becomes a fire. Over time, stability becomes less fragile. Not perfect, but real.

The purpose of this book is not to minimize what bipolar disorder is. The purpose is to help you build a life that is anchored—supported by the right professionals, the right people, and the right daily rhythms—so that this diagnosis does not become your identity.

An anchor does not stop the wind. It does not erase the waves. But it helps you hold your position when conditions change. That is the heart of this book: a set of anchors you can return to—again and again— especially when your mind feels less reliable and your emotions feel bigger than you.

This book assumes one foundational commitment: you will not do this alone. Bipolar disorder is not best managed in isolation. If you have bipolar disorder, the strongest starting point is a psychiatrist—ideally one experienced in bipolar care—who can guide medication management and episode prevention. A therapist can help you build skills, recognize patterns, and repair relationships. A supportive community— faith-based or otherwise—can provide belonging and accountability. And at least one trusted person (family or friend) can learn your early warning signs and help you act early when symptoms rise.

If you do not have all of that in place today, you are not disqualified. You are not behind. Consider this book an invitation to build your foundation step by step. We will keep coming back to one question: What makes stability more likely for your brain?

You will notice that this book treats sleep and daily rhythm with unusual seriousness. That is intentional. For many people with bipolar disorder, sleep disruption is not just inconvenient—it is destabilizing. Protecting sleep is not a personality preference. It is part of treatment. We will also talk about triggers, early warning signs, and what it means to create a contingency plan with your psychiatrist and therapist for the times when your usual tools are not enough.

One more important truth: relapse is not the same as failure. Episodes are not moral verdicts. If you have an episode, it is not proof that you are hopeless. It is evidence that your brain is under strain—and it is information you can use to adjust your plan. Over time, many people grow in self-trust: not because they never struggle, but because they learn how to return to their anchors sooner.

Chapter 1
You Are Not Your Diagnosis

Anchor 1: Identity - You are not your diagnosis.

If you have bipolar disorder, there is a good chance you have tried to explain yourself in a hundred different ways.

Maybe you have told someone, "I'm just stressed."
Maybe you have said, "I'm fine," when you weren't.
Maybe you have tried to make jokes so people would not see how scared you felt.
Maybe you have blamed yourself for being "too much" or "not enough."
Maybe you have quietly wondered if the people you love would be better off without you.

If any of that is familiar, I want you to hear this clearly at the very beginning:

You are not your diagnosis.

A diagnosis is a description of a pattern. It is not a verdict on your worth.
A diagnosis can guide treatment. It cannot define your identity.

And yet, when you have lived through episodes—especially if episodes have cost you relationships, money, jobs, reputation, or peace—it can feel like bipolar disorder is the loudest thing about you. It can feel like you are walking around with a warning label attached to your name.

This chapter is the first anchor for the entire book: separating "who you are" from "what you have," so you can build stability without shame.

Because shame is heavy. And shame is not a treatment plan.

Two truths we will hold together

This book will ask you to hold two truths at the same time—without minimizing either one.

Truth #1: Bipolar disorder is serious.
It is a brain-based medical condition that affects how mood, energy, sleep, motivation, and thinking speed are regulated. (Miklowitz, 2008)

Truth #2: You can live a meaningful, stable life with bipolar disorder.
Not by pretending it is not real, but by treating it with the seriousness it deserves and building supports that make stability more likely. (Frank et al., 2005; Miklowitz et al., 2007)

Some people try to hold only the first truth. They live in fear and self-surveillance, as if one mistake will ruin everything.

Other people try to hold only the second truth. They minimize the illness, skip treatment, and end up blindsided when symptoms return.

Anchored living is holding both:
"This is real—and I can build well."

The story bipolar disorder tries to tell you

Bipolar disorder often comes with a story—a narrative your mind repeats when you look at your life.

It might sound like:
- "I'm unstable."
- "I can't be trusted."
- "I'm a burden."
- "I ruin everything."
- "I'm too much for people."
- "I'm not safe to love."

Sometimes that story gets reinforced by other people—especially people who do not understand the illness, or people who are speaking from their own pain. When you have hurt someone or scared someone during an episode, it makes sense that you would internalize their fear and turn it into a permanent identity.

But the presence of a story does not make it true.

Here is what we can say with clarity:

Bipolar disorder can influence what you feel, what seems urgent, what seems possible, and how fast your mind moves. [Miklowitz, 2008] It can shift sleep and circadian rhythm in ways that affect regulation. [Miklowitz, 2008] It can affect risk perception, impulsivity, and judgment during episodes. [Miklowitz, 2008]

That matters, because it means you cannot "willpower" your way out of every state shift.
And it also matters because it means your worst moments are not a complete picture of who you are.

You are not the illness.
You are a person living with an illness.

Why shame makes everything worse

Many people with bipolar disorder learn to live in a loop that looks like this:

1) Symptoms rise.
2) Life gets chaotic.
3) Consequences follow.
4) Shame floods in.
5) Shame leads to secrecy, isolation, or stubborn independence.
6) Isolation makes symptoms worse.
7) The cycle repeats.

Shame feels like it is doing something useful. It feels like punishment that might prevent the next episode. But shame does not stabilize the brain. Shame does not improve sleep. Shame does not make treatment easier. Shame usually makes you hide—and hiding makes the illness louder.

Shame also tends to distort your memory. It convinces you that your entire life is your worst week. It takes the most dysregulated season of your mind and calls it "the real you."

But stability is not built through self-hatred. Stability is built through truth, support, and consistent care.

A new definition of personal responsibility

Here is a framing that can change everything:

Bipolar disorder is not your fault.
And it is your responsibility to treat it. (Frank et al., 2005; Miklowitz et al., 2007)

Responsibility does not mean you can prevent every episode.
Responsibility means you stop leaving your future to chance.
Responsibility means you build supports while you are well, so that when you are not well you are not alone with the consequences.

Responsibility means you do not make bipolar disorder your identity—but you do make stability your priority.

If you have ever felt trapped between two terrible options—either denying the illness or drowning in it—there is a third way:

Take the illness seriously without taking shame as your identity.

What this book will not do

This book will not shame you.
It will not minimize bipolar disorder.
It will not suggest that faith, mindset, or positive thinking can replace medical care.

It will not ask you to do this alone.

Bipolar disorder is a serious medical condition. Evidence-informed guidelines emphasize long-term treatment planning, monitoring, and support. [Frank et al., 2005; Miklowitz et al., 2007] The most stable outcomes tend to grow when people build a foundation that includes specialty psychiatric care, therapy, reliable supports, and daily rhythms that protect sleep and regulation. [Frank et al., 2005; Miklowitz et al., 2007]

In other words: anchors.

The first anchor: separating identity from symptoms

Before we talk about routines, warning signs, relapse prevention, or contingency plans, we have to name the foundation.

You are not your diagnosis.
You are not your symptoms.
You are not your worst episode.
You are not your best day, either.

You are a whole person.

And if you can hold that truth, you will be able to build the rest of this book without self-erasure.

Because the goal is not to become someone else.
The goal is to become more consistently yourself—by protecting your brain, your relationships, and your future.

What to do when you do not feel like yourself

Some days you will feel clear and steady.
Other days you may feel like your mind is speeding up, sinking down, or tightening into urgent panic.

When you feel that shift, this is a simple phrase to keep nearby:

"This is a state. I will not make identity decisions inside a state."

A state can change.
A state can be treated.
A state can pass.

Your identity is bigger than a state.

Where we are going next

In Chapter 2, we will frame bipolar disorder as a brain health condition in clear, compassionate language— so you can understand what is happening without turning it into shame. (Miklowitz, 2008)

Understanding is not labeling yourself.
Understanding is building a path to stability.

Take five minutes. Answer quickly. No perfection required.

1) When you think about bipolar disorder, what parts feel most tangled up with your sense of identity?

____

____

2) Where do you notice shame showing up most strongly—relationships, work, faith, or self-talk?

____

____

3) If responsibility means "building supports" instead of "forcing control," what is one support you want to strengthen first?
(psychiatrist / therapist / sleep / routine / community / trusted support)

____

____

4) What is one sentence you want to remember the next time symptoms try to define you?

21

____

____

Chapter 2
Understanding Bipolar Disorder as a Brain Health Condition

Anchor 2: Understanding - This is a brain health condition with patterns.

You deserve language for what you live with.

Not labels that make you feel judged.
Not clichés that reduce you to "mood swings."
Not spiritual explanations that ignore biology.
Not medical explanations that ignore your humanity.

Clear language is a stabilizer because it reduces confusion and shame.

So in this chapter we are going to do something simple but powerful:
we will frame bipolar disorder as a brain health condition, and we will name what that means—
practically, compassionately, and with respect for the seriousness of the illness. (Miklowitz, 2008)

Why this framing matters

When people do not understand bipolar disorder, they often interpret symptoms as character.

They call it:
- laziness (when depression makes functioning

harder)
- selfishness (when mania becomes impulsive)
- irresponsibility (when decisions change quickly)
- drama (when emotions become intense)
- inconsistency (when energy rises and falls)

But bipolar disorder is not primarily a problem of character.
It is a problem of regulation. (Miklowitz, 2008)

When regulation is disrupted, it affects:
- mood intensity
- energy and drive
- sleep and circadian rhythm
- thinking speed and focus
- impulse control and risk tolerance (Miklowitz, 2008)

This is one reason you can feel like "two versions" of yourself exist.
You are still you—but your brain state is shifting.
(Miklowitz, 2008)

Understanding this does not excuse harm.
It does not erase accountability.
But it does help you stop confusing symptoms with identity.

Bipolar disorder is not "being emotional"

Everyone has emotions.
Bipolar disorder is different because it involves

episodes—state changes that last long enough and are severe enough to impair functioning or create significant risk. (Miklowitz, 2008)

In the DSM-5-TR, bipolar disorders are defined by patterns that include manic episodes, hypomanic episodes, and depressive episodes, and by the impact these episodes have on functioning. (Miklowitz, 2008)

In plain language:
bipolar disorder is not simply "having big feelings."
It is your brain shifting into a different gear—and staying there longer than is healthy or safe. (Miklowitz, 2008)

A practical picture: the thermostat metaphor

Think of emotional regulation like a thermostat.

Most people's nervous systems adjust temperature gradually:
they get stressed, then settle; they get excited, then return to baseline.

In bipolar disorder, the thermostat is more vulnerable to getting bumped.
Sometimes it gets bumped upward (hypomania/mania).
Sometimes it gets bumped downward (depression).
Sometimes it gets pulled in two directions at once (mixed states). (Miklowitz, 2008)

The goal of treatment is not to remove all emotion.
The goal is to make the thermostat more stable, less
reactive, and easier to reset.

What treatment is actually trying to do

Evidence-informed clinical guidelines emphasize that
bipolar disorder is typically managed with an ongoing
plan that includes pharmacotherapy, monitoring, and
psychosocial supports. (Frank et al., 2005; Miklowitz et al., 2007)

In practical terms, your plan aims to:
- reduce episode frequency (fewer episodes)
- reduce episode severity (less intense episodes)
- shorten episode duration (episodes end sooner)
- reduce episode cost (less fallout)
- improve functioning and quality of life (Frank et al., 2005;
Miklowitz et al., 2007)

This is why we talk about "anchors."
Anchors do not guarantee that storms will never
come.
Anchors reduce how far you drift when storms arrive.

Sleep is not a lifestyle choice; it is a clinical variable

If you have bipolar disorder, sleep is not optional in
the way culture treats it.

For many people with bipolar disorder, sleep
disruption is both:
- a destabilizer (it can contribute to episodes), and

- an early warning sign (it can signal a shift is beginning). ^(Frank et al., 2005; Miklowitz et al., 2007; American Psychiatric Association, 2022)

Sleep disturbance is widely discussed as clinically important in bipolar disorder and has major implications for treatment planning. ^(American Psychiatric Association, 2022)

In other words:
sleep is not only "self-care."
For many people, sleep is part of the medical plan.
(Frank et al., 2005; Miklowitz et al., 2007; American Psychiatric Association, 2022)

You will see sleep return again and again in this book—not because we want to control you, but because sleep often protects you.

Circadian rhythm: the "internal clock" that supports stability

Circadian rhythm is the body's internal timing system—your built-in clock for sleep, alertness, hormones, and daily rhythm.

In bipolar disorder, rhythm dysregulation is a major theme in both clinical and research literature. ^(Miklowitz et al., 2007; McCarthy et al., 2021)

This is one reason rhythm-based approaches, such as interpersonal and social rhythm therapy (IPSRT), focus on stabilizing daily routines (wake time, sleep time, meals, activity, and social rhythms). (Miklowitz et al., 2007)

A practical takeaway:
your brain often does better when your days are more predictable than the average person's days.

That is not weakness.
That is an accommodation for a real condition.
And accommodations keep people well.

Why you may doubt your diagnosis (and why that is common)

Many people with bipolar disorder have seasons of doubt.

They think:
- "Maybe it was just stress."
- "Maybe I was just young."
- "Maybe I am making excuses."
- "Maybe I don't really have this."

Doubt is common for two reasons:

1) When you are well, you may not be able to remember how severe the episode felt.
The human brain has trouble recalling states we are not currently in.

2) Some symptoms can overlap with other conditions (anxiety, ADHD, trauma, substance use, sleep

disorders).
That is why accurate diagnosis and specialty care
matter. (Frank et al., 2005; Miklowitz et al., 2007)

The goal of this book is not to convince you you
"have bipolar disorder."
The goal is to help you build stability if bipolar
disorder is part of your reality—and to encourage you
to pursue careful evaluation and treatment.

The "treat it like diabetes" frame—without minimizing complexity

A helpful way to reduce shame is to compare bipolar
disorder to other chronic, treatable conditions.

If a person has diabetes, they usually need:
- medical care
- medication (sometimes insulin)
- monitoring
- consistent habits (food, activity, sleep)
- education
- support

Diabetes does not become someone's identity.
It becomes something they manage.

Bipolar disorder is different in many ways, but the
principle holds:
it is a serious condition that often requires a long-
term plan. (Frank et al., 2005; Miklowitz et al., 2007)

When you treat bipolar disorder with seriousness and consistency, many people experience improved stability and quality of life. (Frank et al., 2005; Miklowitz et al., 2007)

What stability looks like in real life

Stability does not mean:
- never feeling sad
- never feeling excited
- never having a hard day
- never needing help
- never having symptoms again

Stability often means:
- you notice shifts sooner
- you respond earlier
- you protect sleep and rhythm more consistently
(American Psychiatric Association, 2022; Miklowitz et al., 2007)

- you keep your care team engaged (Frank et al., 2005; Miklowitz et al., 2007)

- you reduce the fallout when symptoms rise (Frank et al., 2005; Miklowitz et al., 2007)

- you return to baseline more quickly

A stable life is not a perfect life.
It is a life with fewer spirals, shorter spirals, and more support inside the spirals.

A word about spirituality (optional, not required)

Because you are reading a book written by a Doctor in Ministry, I want to name this carefully.

Spiritual support can be deeply stabilizing when it is healthy:
- it reduces isolation
- it provides meaning and community
- it strengthens hope
- it supports moral and relational repair

But spiritual care is not a replacement for psychiatric care.

Bipolar disorder is a medical condition, and responsible support honors that. (Frank et al., 2005; Miklowitz et al., 2007)

If faith is part of your life, we will treat it as a resource—not a weapon.

If faith is not part of your life, you are still fully welcome here.

The anchors in this book are built to work for you either way.

Where we are going next

Now that we have named bipolar disorder as a brain health condition, Chapter 3 becomes clearer:
you need a team, not just a willpower strategy.

In Chapter 3 we will talk about building your care team—psychiatry, therapy, and support people—and what it looks like to "anchor yourself for success." (Frank et al., 2005; Miklowitz et al., 2007)

Anchor Check — Chapter 2 ^(Frank et al., 2005)

Choose one (circle it):

1) The hardest part of the brain-health framing for me to accept is:

A) "This is medical"

B) "I need long-term care"

C) "Sleep matters more than I want it to"

D) "My identity is bigger than my symptoms"

E) Other: _______________________________

Write two sentences:

1) When I notice myself sliding into shame, I want to remember:

____

____

2) One practical way I can treat bipolar disorder like a serious condition (without making it my identity) is:

____

____

Optional (if you have support people):
What is one sentence you wish your closest people understood about bipolar disorder as a regulation condition?

____

____

Chapter 3
Your Care Team — Psychiatry, Therapy, and Support

Anchor 3: Team - I do not manage this alone.

If bipolar disorder is a brain health condition, then stability is not a solo project. (Frank et al., 2005; Miklowitz et al., 2007)

This is one of the hardest and most freeing shifts you can make:

you stop trying to outrun bipolar disorder with willpower, and you start building a care team that can hold you steady in seasons when your brain cannot hold itself steady.

You may have learned, through pain, that when your mind "spins out," the cost is not only internal. It can ripple into:
- relationships
- finances
- work and reputation
- legal trouble
- physical safety
- spiritual stability and hope

That is why this chapter is not optional.
It is the foundation for optimizing life with bipolar disorder:

you anchor yourself for success by building a team, a plan, and a support structure that can carry weight.

This chapter will be direct, because bipolar disorder is serious.
And it will be compassionate, because needing care is not shame.

The goal of a care team

A strong care team does four things:

1) It reduces relapse risk by supporting long-term treatment planning. (Frank et al., 2005; Miklowitz et al., 2007)
2) It helps you identify warning signs sooner and respond earlier. (Frank et al., 2005; Miklowitz et al., 2007; Harvey, 2008; Perry et al., 1999)

3) It improves functioning and quality of life by strengthening coping skills and daily rhythms. (Frank et al., 2005; Miklowitz et al., 2007; Miklowitz et al., 2007; Rea et al., 2003)

4) It protects you during escalation by making contingency steps clear. (Frank et al., 2005; Miklowitz et al., 2007)

In other words, a care team does not just "help you talk about your feelings."
A care team helps you build a life that does not collapse every time symptoms rise.

Care Team Starter List

If this book had one non-negotiable recommendation, it would be this:

work with a psychiatrist (or psychiatric prescriber) who is experienced in bipolar disorder. (Frank et al., 2005; Miklowitz et al., 2007)

A general medical doctor can be an important part of your overall health. But bipolar disorder is complex and often requires specialty knowledge and close monitoring. (Frank et al., 2005; Miklowitz et al., 2007)

A psychiatrist helps you with:
- diagnostic clarity
- medication selection and adjustments
- monitoring for side effects and risks
- relapse prevention planning
- rapid response when symptoms escalate (Frank et al., 2005; Miklowitz et al., 2007)

It is common to want to step away from psychiatric care when you feel better.
That is also when relapse prevention is built.

Stability is not only what you do in crisis.
Stability is what you maintain in calm seasons.

A word about medication (direct and respectful)

Medication can be life-changing for many people with bipolar disorder. (Frank et al., 2005; Miklowitz et al., 2007)
Medication is not a spiritual failure.
Medication is not weakness.
Medication is not "cheating."

Medication is one part of treating a brain-based condition.

Some people have strong feelings about medication because of side effects, past bad experiences, or fear of losing their personality. Those concerns deserve to be taken seriously and discussed with your psychiatrist, not hidden in shame. (Frank et al., 2005; Miklowitz et al., 2007)

One of the most important skills you can build is honest collaboration:

- "This medication helps, but I am struggling with side effects."

- "I am worried about weight, sleep, or emotional flattening."

- "I need a plan I can actually stay consistent with."
(Frank et al., 2005; Miklowitz et al., 2007)

Your psychiatrist cannot help you adjust what they do not know.

A therapist who walks with you through real life

Psychiatry treats the biology.
Therapy helps you build the life systems that protect the biology.

Evidence-informed guidelines and research support psychosocial interventions as important adjuncts to medication for many people with bipolar disorder. (Frank et al., 2005; Miklowitz et al., 2007; Perry et al., 1999; Colom et al., 2003; Yatham et al., 2018)

A good therapist can help you:
- map your episode signature (how bipolar shows up for you)
- identify early warning signs and triggers (Harvey, 2008; Perry et al., 1999)

- build routines and boundaries that protect sleep and rhythm (Miklowitz et al., 2007; Rea et al., 2003)
- reduce shame and increase accountability
- repair relationships after episodes (National Institute for Health and Care Excellence, 2014; Frank, 2007)

- strengthen decision guardrails to reduce fallout (Frank et al., 2005; Miklowitz et al., 2007)

What you want is not only insight.
You want integration: a therapist who helps you turn awareness into a plan.

What to look for in a therapist

You are not looking for a perfect therapist. You are looking for a therapist who is:
- stable and consistent
- respectful of bipolar disorder as medical
- willing to coordinate with psychiatry

Some therapies focus heavily on the past. That can be valuable. But with bipolar disorder, you also need a therapist who can help you build the present:
sleep protection, rhythm, relationships, relapse prevention, and contingency planning.

Support people who understand the diagnosis

Bipolar disorder often isolates people.
Not only because of symptoms, but because of fear of how others will respond.

But isolation increases risk.

Family and support-focused approaches highlight the value of informed support systems that can help reduce relapse burden and improve outcomes. (National Institute for Health and Care Excellence, 2014; Frank, 2007)

Support people are not meant to "monitor" you like you are a problem.
They are meant to help you stay anchored—especially when your mind is convincing you that you do not need anyone.

Healthy support looks like:
- calm honesty
- predictable connection
- respect for boundaries
- willingness to follow an agreed plan (not improvise in crisis) (National Institute for Health and Care Excellence, 2014; Frank, 2007)

If you have been hurt by controlling or shaming
support, it makes sense that you feel resistant.
That is why we define support carefully in this book:
support is not control.
Support is partnership.

A community that does not shame you

This book is not strictly faith-based, but it is written
by someone whose training includes spiritual care.
So I will say this plainly:

Community can be stabilizing when it is healthy.
Community becomes harmful when it is shaming.

Whether your community is faith-based or not, look
for people who:
- take bipolar disorder seriously as a medical
condition
- respect treatment and do not discourage it
- support stable rhythms and boundaries (not
constant intensity)
- respond to relapse with compassion and
accountability, not gossip or condemnation

A healthy community does not replace psychiatry.
It supports your humanity while psychiatry supports
your brain. (Frank et al., 2005; Miklowitz et al., 2007)

How your team works together (coordination, not chaos)

One of the most stabilizing things you can do is create shared language across your supports.

That includes:
- how you describe your early warning signs
- what counts as yellow zone vs. red zone
- what you want support people to do (and not do)
- how you contact clinicians early
- what your emergency plan is if you need a higher level of care [Frank et al., 2005; Miklowitz et al., 2007]

When supporters do not have shared language, they panic.
When they panic, they argue.
When they argue, things escalate.

Shared language reduces escalation.

This is why later chapters and appendices include:
- warning sign mapping
- anchor checks
- a contingency plan worksheet
- scripts for appointments and support conversations

We are building a system that works even when your nervous system does not.

"But I don't have money for this" (a compassionate reality check)

Some readers will think, I cannot afford a psychiatrist and a therapist and support systems.
I want to acknowledge that access is real, and barriers are real.

Even with barriers, you can still work toward the principle:
do not try to manage bipolar disorder alone.

Depending on your location and resources, "team building" might include:
- community mental health clinics
- sliding-scale therapy
- telepsychiatry
- peer support groups
- case management
- trusted support people who are willing to learn and follow a plan

The shape of your team may vary.
The need for a team does not.

The most important question of this chapter

If your brain state changed tomorrow—up, down, or mixed—would you have enough support to stay safe and reduce fallout? (Frank et al., 2005; Miklowitz et al., 2007)

If the answer is "no," you are not behind.
You are simply at the next step.

This chapter is your permission slip to take your condition seriously and build the supports you deserve.

Where we are going next

In Chapter 4, we move from "team building" to "support in real life":
how to help the people around you understand bipolar disorder, how to set boundaries that protect stability, and how to build community that supports your life rather than complicates it. (National Institute for Health and Care Excellence, 2014; Frank, 2007)

Anchor Check — Chapter 3 (Miklowitz et al., 2007)

Build Your Team

Choose one step you can take in the next 14 days:

1) Psychiatry:
☐ I will schedule an appointment (or follow-up) with a psychiatrist experienced in bipolar disorder. (Frank et al., 2005; Miklowitz et al., 2007)

2) Therapy:
☐ I will identify and contact one therapist who can support relapse prevention planning (warning signs, rhythms, repair). (Frank et al., 2005; Miklowitz et al., 2007)

3) Support:
☐ I will choose one trusted person and say: "I'm building a stability plan. Would you be willing to be part of my support circle?" (National Institute for Health and Care Excellence, 2014; Frank, 2007)

Write one sentence you can use with yourself:
"When I feel like I should do this alone, I will remember: _______________________________."

Optional (if you have clinicians):
What is one question you want to ask your psychiatrist or therapist at the next appointment?

____

Chapter 4
Community, Family, and the People Who Help You Stay Anchored

Anchor 4: Support - I build a wise circle and healthy boundaries.

One of the hardest parts of bipolar disorder is that it can change how connected you feel to other people.

When you are depressed, you may feel:
- like you are a burden
- like no one understands
- like disappearing would protect everyone

When you are up, you may feel:
- like you do not need anyone
- like people slow you down
- like limits feel intolerable

When you are mixed or agitated, you may feel:
- easily provoked
- suspicious of others' motives
- desperate for relief and frustrated with help

These states can pull you toward isolation or conflict—sometimes both at the same time. (Miklowitz, 2008; Frank et al., 2005)

This chapter is about building the kind of community and family support that protects stability without turning your life into a surveillance project.

Not everyone is safe.
Not everyone is wise.
Not everyone deserves access to your inner world.

But you do need people.

Bipolar disorder is serious, and evidence-informed approaches recognize that informed family and social support can improve outcomes and reduce relapse burden. (National Institute for Health and Care Excellence, 2014; Frank, 2007; Perry et al., 1999)

Why support matters (and why it can also feel complicated)

Many people with bipolar disorder have been hurt by "support."

Support that looked like:
- control
- criticism
- minimizing ("Just snap out of it.")
- spiritual bypass ("Just pray harder.")
- fear-driven lectures
- gossip
- punishments disguised as love

If you have experienced that, your resistance makes sense.

The problem is that the illness often uses that pain to argue for isolation:
"People only make it worse. I can do this alone."

But isolation is not neutral. Isolation can increase risk, delay help-seeking, and make spirals more expensive. (Frank et al., 2005; Miklowitz et al., 2007; National Institute for Health and Care Excellence, 2014; Frank, 2007)

So the goal is not "let everyone in."
The goal is "build a wise circle."

Your support circle: inner, middle, and outer

One way to make support less chaotic is to think in circles:

Inner Circle (1–3 people)
These are the people who:
- know your diagnosis
- know your warning signs
- know your plan
- can speak up when you are shifting
- are allowed to help initiate next steps (with your consent)

This circle is not about the number. It is about reliability.

Middle Circle (a few more people)
These are people who support you emotionally and practically, but do not need every detail.
They may know you live with bipolar disorder, but they are not the ones making crisis calls.

Outer Circle (community)
These are people who help you feel human: neighbors, faith community, small group, coworkers, friends, peer support.
They provide connection and meaning, not clinical monitoring.

This structure protects you from oversharing and protects others from being overloaded.

How to choose the right support people

The best support people are not necessarily the people who love you the most.
They are the people who can stay grounded when things get intense. (National Institute for Health and Care Excellence, 2014; Frank, 2007)

Look for people who:
- can be calm under stress
- do not panic easily
- do not shame you
- respect clinical care and do not discourage it (Frank et al., 2005; Miklowitz et al., 2007)

- can be direct without being cruel

- can follow a plan (instead of improvising from fear)
- can keep confidence and avoid gossip

A simple question to ask yourself:
When my emotions rise, does this person become more stable—or more chaotic?

Choose stability.

What supporters need from you (and what you need from them)

Healthy support is mutual clarity.

Supporters need:
- permission to name what they see (without fear of retaliation)
- clear boundaries (what is their role and what is not)
- a plan they can follow
- confidence that you will return to repair if things go sideways [National Institute for Health and Care Excellence, 2014; Frank, 2007]

You need:
- calm, honest feedback
- predictable connection
- respect (not infantilization)
- a shared language for early warning signs and escalation [Frank et al., 2005; Miklowitz et al., 2007; Harvey, 2008]
- practical help when symptoms rise (meals, rides, childcare, reduced stimulation)
- protection from late-night conflict and impulsive

decision spirals (American Psychiatric Association, 2022; Miklowitz et al., 2007)

Support is not "fixing you."
Support is helping you stay tethered to your plan when your brain state tries to rewrite it.

The most important skill: giving permission while you are well

One of the best things you can do for your relationships is to decide, while you are stable, what you want others to do when you are not stable. (Frank et al., 2005; Miklowitz et al., 2007)

This is what reduces betrayal feelings later.
Supporters can say:
"We are following the plan you made when you were well." (Frank et al., 2005; Miklowitz et al., 2007)

That sentence protects trust.

Practical permissions you can give (choose what fits):
- "If you notice my sleep is slipping, please tell me directly and calmly." (American Psychiatric Association, 2022; Harvey, 2008)

- "If I have not slept for two nights and I say I'm fine, please encourage me to contact my psychiatrist." (Frank et al., 2005; Miklowitz et al., 2007; Harvey, 2008)

- "If I am escalating, please do not argue with me.

Help me reduce stimulation and follow the plan." (National Institute for Health and Care Excellence, 2014; Frank, 2007)

- "If you are concerned, ask me one simple question: 'Have you slept? Are you taking meds? Are you connected to care?'" (Frank et al., 2005; Miklowitz et al., 2007; American Psychiatric Association, 2022)

Boundaries that protect stability (and protect love)

Boundaries are not rejection. They are protection.

Some boundaries that help many people with bipolar disorder:
- No major conversations after a certain hour (especially after wind-down starts). (American Psychiatric Association, 2022)

- No ultimatums during yellow/red zone.
- No spending or decision debates when sleep is disrupted. (American Psychiatric Association, 2022)
- Support people are allowed to take breaks from conflict (stepping away is not abandonment).
- We return to discussions when both people are regulated.

Boundaries keep relationships from becoming collateral damage.

Family pain is real: moving from blame to pattern

If your family has been impacted by episodes, some people may carry fear, trauma, or resentment.

That does not make them bad.
It means the experience was costly.

Family-focused work emphasizes education,
communication skills, and relapse prevention
planning to reduce conflict and improve stability.
(National Institute for Health and Care Excellence, 2014; Frank, 2007)

A gentle but important truth:
You cannot heal family trust with one apology.
You heal it through consistency and repair over time.

That is why Chapter 9 is coming later.
But in this chapter, we start the foundation:
stable communication, boundaries, and shared
planning.

If your family is unsafe or unwilling

Some readers do not have supportive family.
Some families are abusive, addicted, controlling, or
deeply shaming.
Some families refuse to believe the diagnosis or refuse
treatment support.

If that is you:
you are not disqualified from stability.

Your support circle can be built outside your family:
- friends
- mentors
- peer support groups

- therapy relationships
- faith community (if safe)
- chosen family

The goal is not "family closeness at all costs."
The goal is "support that protects health."

A simple script to invite someone into your inner circle

Here is language you can adapt:

"I'm working on stability with my care team. Bipolar disorder is a medical condition for me, and I'm building a plan to reduce the cost when symptoms rise. I'm not asking you to fix me. I'm asking if you would be willing to be someone I can be honest with—someone who can notice early warning signs and help me follow the plan I made while I'm well."
(National Institute for Health and Care Excellence, 2014; Frank, 2007)

If they say no, that is information.
If they say yes, follow with:
"Here is what helps. Here is what does not help. Here is what I want you to do if you are concerned."

Clarity is love.

Where we are going next

In Chapter 5, we will map your "episode signature"—the specific pattern of how bipolar shows up for you—so you and your support circle can recognize shifts sooner and respond with less panic. (Frank et al., 2005; Harvey, 2008)

Pick one action for this week:

1) Circle-building:
Write the names of your circles (even if some are blank):
Inner Circle (1–3):

____

Middle Circle:

____

Outer Circle / Community:

____

2) One boundary that protects stability:
Complete the sentence:
"To protect my stability and my relationships, I will not have major conversations after ___________."
(American Psychiatric Association, 2022)

3) One permission you will give while well:
Complete the sentence:
"If you notice ________________________, I give you permission to say it out loud and encourage me to follow my plan." (Frank et al., 2005; Miklowitz et al., 2007; Harvey, 2008)

Optional (if you feel ready):

Who is one person you could invite into your inner circle using the script in this chapter?

____

____

Chapter 5
Your Episode Signature — How Your Bipolar Shows Up

Anchor 5: Signature - I know my pattern.

If you have lived with bipolar disorder for any length of time, you have probably asked yourself a question that sounds like this:

"Why does this keep happening to me?"

Sometimes that question carries shame.
Sometimes it carries fear.
Sometimes it carries exhaustion.

But there is another way to approach it—one that is steadier and more hopeful:

"What does my pattern look like?"

Because bipolar disorder has patterns, and you can learn yours. (Frank et al., 2005; Harvey, 2008)

A diagnosis gives a category.
Your episode signature gives a map.

This chapter is about building that map.

What is an "episode signature"?

Your episode signature is the specific way bipolar disorder shows up in your life.

Two people can both have bipolar disorder and look very different:
- one person may trend toward depression with rare hypomania
- another may have clearer manic episodes
- another may experience mixed states
- one may become irritable and agitated
- another may become euphoric and impulsive

The diagnosis names the condition.
The signature names your version of it. (Miklowitz, 2008)

Your signature includes:
- your most common episode types (up, down, mixed)
- your early warning signs (what changes first)
- your triggers (what pushes you closer to shifting)
- your "tells" (what other people notice)
- your common fallout areas (money, relationships, work, sleep)
- what helps you return sooner (Frank et al., 2005; Miklowitz et al., 2007; Harvey, 2008)

When you know your signature, you can act earlier—and early action often changes outcomes. (Frank et al., 2005; Miklowitz et al., 2007; Harvey, 2008)

Why mapping matters (and why it's not "self-labeling")

Some readers resist mapping because they worry it will make them obsess.

That is a fair concern.
But mapping is not about staring at yourself all day.
Mapping is about reducing surprises.

Many people do not get hurt most by the episode itself.
They get hurt by the surprise of the episode:
the confusion, the denial, the delayed response, the chaos.

A signature gives you earlier clarity.
And clarity is protective.

The three common states to understand (in plain language)

This is not a diagnostic checklist (that belongs with clinicians).
This is practical language to help you notice patterns.
(Miklowitz, 2008)

Down-shift (depressive state)
Often includes:
- low energy, heavy body
- slower thinking
- low motivation

- hopelessness or numbness
- withdrawing from people
- changes in sleep (too much or disrupted)
- shame and self-criticism becoming louder [Miklowitz, 2008]

Your down-shift signature might be quieter than people expect.
Sometimes the most dangerous depression is silent.

Up-shift (hypomania/mania)
Often includes:
- less sleep with more energy
- faster thinking
- increased confidence
- increased talking or activity
- impulsivity (spending, sex, work, plans)
- irritability or agitation (not always euphoria)
- feeling like limits are intolerable [Miklowitz, 2008]

A key point:
Many people miss early up-shift signs because it can feel good at first.
It can feel like "I'm finally me."
That is why signature work matters.

Mixed state (up and down at the same time)
Often includes:
- agitation plus despair
- energy plus hopelessness

- restlessness plus sadness
- racing thoughts plus dark thoughts
- feeling trapped, reactive, or desperate for relief
(Miklowitz, 2008)

Mixed states can be especially risky.
They are one reason contingency planning matters.
(Frank et al., 2005; Miklowitz et al., 2007)

Your first question: What changes first?

For many people with bipolar disorder, the first
change is not mood.
It is sleep. (American Psychiatric Association, 2022; Miklowitz et al., 2007)

Or it is speed:
- talking faster
- thinking faster
- moving faster
- taking on more
- feeling urgent

Or it is social rhythm:
- staying up later
- skipping meals
- missing routines
- changing structure suddenly (Miklowitz et al., 2007; Rea et al., 2003)

A powerful mapping question:
"What is the earliest, smallest sign that I am shifting?"
(Harvey, 2008)

This sign is gold.
It is the difference between a yellow zone response
and a red zone crisis.

The "tells": what other people notice

You may not be the first person to notice your shift.
That is not an insult.
It is a feature of how episodes work.

People close to you may notice:
- a change in sleep schedule
- a change in tone (more sharp, more intense, more
withdrawn)
- a change in volume or speed
- a change in spending or online activity
- a change in risk tolerance
- a change in how you respond to feedback [National
Institute for Health and Care Excellence, 2014; Frank, 2007]

This is why Chapter 4 mattered.
You need at least one person who can tell you the
truth without shaming you.

A practical exercise:
Ask one trusted person:
"When you think I'm shifting, what do you notice
first?" [National Institute for Health and Care Excellence, 2014; Frank, 2007]

Write it down.
Do not argue.
Treat it as data.

Triggers versus warning signs (do not confuse them)

A trigger is something that pushes.
A warning sign is something that signals you are already moving. [Harvey, 2008]

Triggers might include:
- sleep loss
- conflict
- big life changes
- grief
- travel/time zone shifts
- substance use
- seasonal changes
- overwork or overstimulation [Frank et al., 2005; Miklowitz et al., 2007; American Psychiatric Association, 2022]

Warning signs are the internal and external clues that your state is shifting:
- reduced sleep
- increased speed
- increased irritability
- increased impulsivity
- withdrawal
- hopelessness

- agitation
- changes in appetite or routine [Harvey, 2008]

You cannot always avoid triggers.
But you can respond to warning signs sooner.

The four categories of your signature map

Use these categories to build your signature. Keep it simple.

1) Sleep signature
- What does sleep look like before an up-shift? [American Psychiatric Association, 2022]

- What does sleep look like before a down-shift? [American Psychiatric Association, 2022]

- What is your "danger threshold" (e.g., less than ___ hours for ___ nights)? [Frank et al., 2005; Miklowitz et al., 2007; Harvey, 2008]

2) Speed signature
- What happens to your thinking speed?
- How does your speech change?
- Do you become more urgent, more confident, more reactive?
- Do you feel like you "cannot slow down"? [Miklowitz, 2008]

3) Social and structure signature
- Do you cancel everything?
- Do you overbook yourself?

- Do you stop eating regular meals?
- Do you stop returning texts?
- Do you start staying up late "just to finish one more thing"? (Miklowitz et al., 2007; Rea et al., 2003)

4) Fallout signature
- Where does bipolar disorder cost you the most? Money? Relationships? Work? Health? Reputation? (Frank et al., 2005; Miklowitz et al., 2007)

This is not about guilt.
This is about protecting the vulnerable places first.

A compassionate warning: do not romanticize your up-shifts

Some people grieve the loss of mania or hypomania. They miss the energy, creativity, confidence, and productivity.

That grief is real.
And it is also dangerous if it leads you to stop protecting sleep or stop treatment.

If you have ever thought,
"I wish I could be that version of me again,"
remember this:
you are remembering the beginning, not the cost.

Signature work helps you remember the whole truth: what starts as energy can become destruction if it escalates. (Frank et al., 2005; Miklowitz et al., 2007)

The goal is not to erase your gifts.
The goal is to protect your life from the part of the
up-shift that becomes expensive.

How to use your signature map with your care team

Bring your signature map to:
- psychiatry appointments
- therapy sessions
- contingency planning conversations [Frank et al., 2005; Miklowitz et al., 2007]

You can say:
"This is what changes first for me.
This is what red zone looks like for me.
This is the earliest point I'm willing to intervene." [Frank et al., 2005; Miklowitz et al., 2007; Harvey, 2008]

That is an empowered patient.
That is anchored living.

Where we are going next

In Chapter 6, we will take your signature map and
turn it into an early-warning plan: what to do in
yellow zone, how to respond before things become
catastrophic, and how to involve your care team
sooner. [Frank et al., 2005; Miklowitz et al., 2007; Harvey, 2008]

Anchor Check — Chapter 5 ^(Miklowitz et al., 2007)

Complete your first draft episode signature map (keep it short).

1) My earliest warning sign is usually (sleep / speed / mood / social rhythm):

____

____

2) My top 3 "up-shift" signs are:

1) ____

2) ____

3) ____

3) My top 3 "down-shift" signs are:

1) ____

2) ____

3) ____

4) My top 2 "mixed / agitation" signs are:

1) _______________________________

2) _______________________________

5) My most expensive fallout area is usually (money / relationships / work / other):

____

____

Optional (high value):
Ask one trusted person: "What do you notice first when I'm shifting?" (National Institute for Health and Care Excellence, 2014; Frank, 2007)

Write their answer here:

____

____

Chapter 6
Early Warning Signs and Triggers — Catching Shifts Early

Anchor 6: Early response - I catch shifts early and act sooner.

If bipolar disorder is a storm system, early warning signs are the radar.

They do not guarantee a storm will hit.
But they give you time.
And time is one of the most powerful resources you have with this diagnosis. (Frank et al., 2005; Miklowitz et al., 2007; Harvey, 2008)

This chapter is about learning the difference between:
- what pushes you (triggers), and
- what signals you are already moving (warning signs). (Harvey, 2008)

When people say, "It came out of nowhere," it usually did not.
It often came with a trail of small clues that were easy to minimize.

This is not about blaming yourself for missing clues.
This is about giving your stable self a way to protect your future self.

Why "catching it early" changes outcomes

A key finding in psychoeducation and relapse-prevention research is that people can be taught to recognize early symptoms and seek treatment sooner, which can reduce relapse-related harm. (Harvey, 2008)

Guidelines also emphasize ongoing monitoring and early intervention as part of long-term management. (Frank et al., 2005; Miklowitz et al., 2007)

In plain language:
earlier action tends to reduce cost.

Early action does not always prevent an episode.
But early action often changes:
- duration (how long it lasts)
- severity (how intense it becomes)
- fallout (how expensive it is)
- safety (how risky it becomes) (Frank et al., 2005; Miklowitz et al., 2007; Harvey, 2008)

Triggers versus warning signs (keep this simple)

Here is the simplest distinction:

A trigger is something that increases vulnerability.
A warning sign is something that tells you vulnerability has turned into movement. (Harvey, 2008)

Triggers can stack quietly for days or weeks.
Warning signs are the "first symptoms" that show the shift is already underway.

Examples of triggers
- sleep loss or irregular schedule (American Psychiatric Association, 2022; Miklowitz et al., 2007)

- travel or time zone shifts
- big life transitions
- conflict or relationship rupture
- grief and anniversaries
- overstimulation (too many commitments, too much social intensity)
- substance use or sudden withdrawal (Frank et al., 2005; Miklowitz et al., 2007)

- stopping medication or inconsistent medication (Frank et al., 2005; Miklowitz et al., 2007)

- seasonal changes
- major hormonal shifts (for some people)

Triggers are not your fault.
But triggers are often your responsibility to plan around.

Examples of warning signs
- sleeping less and not feeling tired (American Psychiatric Association, 2022)

- waking early and unable to return to sleep (American Psychiatric Association, 2022)

- feeling "wired" at night (American Psychiatric Association, 2022)

- increased speed: talking faster, thinking faster, planning more
- irritability rising without a clear reason
- unusual confidence or "destiny" thinking [Miklowitz, 2008]
- impulsive spending or risk-taking
- withdrawing, cancelling, or going quiet
- hopelessness, numbness, or dark thoughts [Miklowitz, 2008]

- agitation, restlessness, or feeling trapped [Miklowitz, 2008]

Warning signs are not moral failures.
They are clinical data.

The #1 warning sign to take seriously: sleep

For many people with bipolar disorder, sleep is both the first domino and the first alarm. [American Psychiatric Association, 2022; Miklowitz et al., 2007]

You may notice:
- trouble falling asleep even when tired
- waking early with a racing mind
- reduced need for sleep
- sleeping but not restoring
- a shifted schedule (staying up later, sleeping later)
- insomnia after overstimulation or conflict [American Psychiatric Association, 2022]

Sleep disruption is so significant in bipolar disorder that it is repeatedly emphasized in clinical discussions and treatment planning. [American Psychiatric Association, 2022]

This is why your "yellow zone" plan often begins with sleep protection.

If you do not take anything else from this chapter, take this:
Sleep changes are worth acting on early.

Your episode signature becomes your warning-sign list

In Chapter 5 you mapped your signature.
Now we make it actionable.

Most people can't track 30 warning signs.
They get overwhelmed and stop.

You want:
- 3–5 early warning signs (yellow zone)
- 3–5 escalation signs (red zone)

Short lists get used.
Long lists get ignored.

Yellow zone: what "early" looks like

Yellow zone is not crisis.
Yellow zone is "pay attention and protect."

Yellow zone might include:
- 1–2 nights of reduced sleep [American Psychiatric Association, 2022; Harvey, 2008]

- increased speed but still some insight
- irritability rising

- mild impulsivity
- noticeable withdrawal
- subtle hopelessness
- change in routines ^(Miklowitz et al., 2007)

Yellow zone is where you have the most leverage.

Red zone: what "tools aren't enough" looks like

Red zone is where:
- insight narrows
- judgment becomes unreliable
- risk increases
- support people may need to step in
- clinical contact becomes urgent ^(Frank et al., 2005; Miklowitz et al., 2007)

Red zone might include:
- severe insomnia or not sleeping ^(American Psychiatric Association, 2022)

- escalating impulsivity (spending, sex, driving, conflict)
- paranoia, loss of reality testing ^(Miklowitz, 2008)
- severe agitation or mixed state distress ^(Miklowitz, 2008)
- suicidal thoughts or self-harm urges ^(Frank et al., 2005; Miklowitz et al., 2007)

- refusing care while symptoms escalate
- loved ones expressing serious concern ^(National Institute for Health and Care Excellence, 2014; Frank, 2007)

Red zone is not the time to negotiate with your symptoms.
Red zone is the time to follow the plan.

The "stacking" effect: why small things suddenly become big

People often ask, "Why did I blow up over something small?"

Sometimes it's because the "small thing" was not the real cause.
It was the final weight on an already overloaded system.

Triggers stack.
Warning signs appear.
Then one more stressor makes everything feel unbearable.

When you understand stacking, you stop blaming your character and start adjusting your load.

A practical yellow zone plan (do this in advance)

Your yellow zone plan should be so simple you can do it when you are tired.

Here is a framework you can adapt (and later we will build this into your contingency plan):

1) Protect sleep immediately. (American Psychiatric Association, 2022; Miklowitz et al., 2007)

2) Reduce stimulation and schedule load. (Frank et al., 2005; Miklowitz et al., 2007)

3) Increase connection (do not isolate). (National Institute for Health and Care Excellence, 2014; Frank, 2007)

4) Notify your care team early if thresholds are met. (Frank et al., 2005; Miklowitz et al., 2007; Harvey, 2008)

5) Activate agreed guardrails (spending limits, no big decisions). (Frank et al., 2005; Miklowitz et al., 2007)

This is not about being controlled.
This is about protecting your life.

When to contact your psychiatrist or therapist (thresholds)

Many people wait too long because they fear being judged, or they do not want to "bother" clinicians.

If you have bipolar disorder, early contact is not bothering.
It is prevention.

A helpful way to decide is to set thresholds while stable, such as:
- sleep less than ___ hours for ___ nights (American Psychiatric Association, 2022; Harvey, 2008)

- racing thoughts + increased speed for ___ days
- rising hopelessness for ___ days
- escalating irritability with conflict patterns
- any safety concern (self-harm, harm to others, inability to function) (Frank et al., 2005; Miklowitz et al., 2007)

76

Your team can help you determine the thresholds that fit your history.

The emotional skill inside early warning work: humility

Early warning work requires a specific kind of courage:
the courage to admit you might be shifting before you "prove it."

Many people delay early action because they want certainty:
- "I don't want to overreact."
- "Maybe it will pass."
- "It's not that bad."

But stability is not built on certainty.
Stability is built on wise response to probability.

If the cost of being wrong is small, act early.
If you protect sleep and reduce load and you were "fine," the result is still healthy.
If you do nothing and you were not fine, the cost can be high.

Where we are going next

In Chapter 7, we take the most powerful anchor in the whole book—sleep and daily rhythms—and build it into a lifestyle that supports long-term stability.
(American Psychiatric Association, 2022; Miklowitz et al., 2007; Rea et al., 2003)

Anchor Check — Chapter 6 ^(Harvey, 2008)

Choose 3 early warning signs and 3 red zone signs.

My 3 yellow zone early warning signs are: ^(Harvey, 2008)

1) ____

2) ____

3) ____

My 3 red zone escalation signs are:

1) ____

2) ____

3) ____

My first yellow zone action will be (one sentence):
(Frank et al., 2005; Miklowitz et al., 2007; American Psychiatric Association, 2022)

____

My clinician contact threshold (fill in):

If I sleep less than _____ hours for _____ nights, I will contact my psychiatrist/therapist. ^(American Psychiatric Association, 2022; Harvey, 2008)

Chapter 7
Sleep and Daily Rhythms — Your Most Powerful Anchor

Anchor 7: Rhythm - I protect sleep and daily rhythms.

If you want one anchor that reliably lowers the cost of bipolar disorder for many people, start here:

Protect sleep.
Protect rhythm.

This chapter is not glamorous. It is not trendy. It is not "hack your life."
It is foundational.

For many people with bipolar disorder, sleep and daily rhythm are not just self-care—they are part of the medical plan. (Frank et al., 2005; Miklowitz et al., 2007; American Psychiatric Association, 2022; Miklowitz et al., 2007; McCarthy et al., 2021; Rea et al., 2003)

When sleep slips, the brain becomes more vulnerable.
When rhythm becomes chaotic, the nervous system loses a key stabilizer.
When those stabilizers are gone, episodes can escalate faster and cost more. (American Psychiatric Association, 2022; Miklowitz et al., 2007)

So we are going to treat sleep and rhythm with respect.

Why sleep is so powerful in bipolar disorder

Sleep influences emotion regulation, cognition, impulse control, stress response, and circadian timing.
In bipolar disorder, sleep disturbance is common and clinically significant, with important therapeutic implications. (American Psychiatric Association, 2022)

Many people notice that their episodes are preceded by:
- less sleep
- delayed sleep time
- fragmented sleep
- waking early with racing thoughts
- feeling "wired" at night (American Psychiatric Association, 2022)

Some people also notice that their depression is tied to hypersomnia or disrupted sleep.
Either way, sleep disruption is not neutral.

When you protect sleep, you are not being boring.
You are being wise.

Rhythm is not rigidity: it is safety

Some readers hear "routines" and feel threatened.
They think:
- "I don't want my life to be controlled."
- "I'm not a child."

- "I'm creative. I need freedom."
- "I can't live like a machine."

Good news:
you do not need to live like a machine.

Rhythm is not perfection.
Rhythm is predictability where it matters most.

Rhythm says:
"I will give my brain what it needs, consistently,
because it does better that way."

Interpersonal and social rhythm therapy (IPSRT) was
designed around the idea that stabilizing daily
rhythms helps address rhythm dysregulation in
bipolar disorder. (Miklowitz et al., 2007)
In other words, rhythm is not a personality
preference—it is a clinical strategy. (Miklowitz et al., 2007; Rea et
al., 2003)

The three rhythm pillars

If you only stabilize three things, stabilize these:

1) Wake time (most important)
2) Bedtime / wind-down window
3) Regular daily anchors (meals, activity, connection)

Many people try to control bedtime first.
But wake time is often the stronger stabilizer.

Wake time: the anchor that trains your brain

A consistent wake time helps regulate circadian rhythm.
It also helps regulate sleep pressure (your body's drive to sleep at night).

Pick a wake time you can keep most days—even on weekends.
If you change it, change it slightly.
The goal is not punishment. The goal is stability.

If you are currently in a depressive season and oversleeping is part of your signature, work on wake time gently and gradually, ideally with your clinician's support. (Frank et al., 2005; Miklowitz et al., 2007)
If you are in an up-shift season and sleeping less is part of your signature, wake time alone will not be enough—you will need additional supports and possibly urgent clinical input. (Frank et al., 2005; Miklowitz et al., 2007; American Psychiatric Association, 2022)

Wind-down: the boundary your brain needs

Many people with bipolar disorder try to "earn" sleep.
They work until they collapse.
They scroll until their eyes hurt.
They argue late at night.
They chase stimulation because quiet feels uncomfortable.

But sleep does not come from forcing.
Sleep comes from creating conditions.

A wind-down window is not a luxury.
It is a boundary that protects your nervous system.

A basic wind-down window includes:
- reducing light and screens
- reducing stimulation and conflict
- calming activities (shower, reading, gentle music)
- repeating the same sequence most nights

You are training your brain: "This is the path to sleep."

What to do when your mind is racing at night

This is one of the most painful experiences in bipolar disorder:
your body is tired, but your mind will not slow down.

Here is a simple response framework:
- do not fight your thoughts
- reduce stimulation
- return to the same calming sequence
- treat it as data, not failure [American Psychiatric Association, 2022]

If racing thoughts + insomnia persist, this is a yellow zone warning sign.
Do not wait until it becomes crisis.
Use your clinician contact thresholds. [Frank et al., 2005; Miklowitz et al., 2007; American Psychiatric Association, 2022; Harvey, 2008]

The "no big conversations at night" rule

Late-night intensity can destabilize sleep and increase conflict cost.
For many people with bipolar disorder, night-time is a vulnerable window.

A stabilizing boundary:
No major conversations after wind-down starts.
No decisions after 9 p.m. (or your chosen time).
No relationship ultimatums in the dark.

This is not avoidance.
This is timing wisdom.

Social rhythm: why your days matter, not just your nights

Sleep is not isolated.
Your day structure influences your night structure.

IPSRT emphasizes the importance of regularity in daily routines (sleep/wake, meals, social activity) because rhythm disruption can destabilize mood.
(Miklowitz et al., 2007; Rea et al., 2003)

In practical terms:
If your days are chaotic, your nights often become chaotic.
If your days are predictable, your nights often become easier.

Daily anchors that help many people:
- regular meals (not skipping)
- movement (even gentle)
- sunlight in the morning
- limited caffeine late in the day
- consistent connection (one text, one call, one check-in)
- a clear end-of-work boundary

Sleep protection is not only for you; it protects the people around you

One of the most loving things you can do for your relationships is protect sleep.

Sleep protection reduces the likelihood of escalation, impulsive decisions, and conflict spirals.
It lowers the "price tag" your loved ones pay when symptoms rise.

This is not about guilt.
It is about shared wellbeing.

When sleep strategies are not enough

Sometimes you can do everything "right" and still not sleep.
That is not failure.
That is information.

If you have bipolar disorder, persistent insomnia can be clinically important and may require prompt medical attention, medication adjustment, or higher-level support. (Frank et al., 2005; Miklowitz et al., 2007; American Psychiatric Association, 2022)

Do not white-knuckle insomnia in isolation.
If you are not sleeping, involve your treatment team.

And if you are moving into red zone, follow the contingency plan.
Chapter 8 is coming for a reason.

A simple 7-day rhythm reset (gentle, realistic)

If you are stable enough to try it, here is a simple reset:

For 7 days:
1) Keep wake time within a 60-minute window.
2) Create a 30–60 minute wind-down window.
3) Reduce caffeine after early afternoon (choose a cutoff time).
4) Move your body gently once a day.
5) Get morning light when possible.
6) Reduce late-night stimulation (especially conflict).
7) Tell one support person, "I'm protecting sleep this week."

The goal is not perfection.
The goal is momentum.

Where we are going next

In Chapter 8, we talk about what happens when your tools are not enough—how to plan for escalation while you are stable, how to keep dignity in crisis, and how to build a contingency plan that protects autonomy. (Frank et al., 2005; Miklowitz et al., 2007)

Anchor Check — Chapter 7 (National Institute for Health and Care Excellence, 2014)

Choose one rhythm anchor to strengthen this week (circle one):

A) Wake time

B) Wind-down window

C) "No big conversations at night" boundary

D) Morning light + gentle movement

E) Caffeine cutoff time

Write your plan in one sentence:
This week, I will protect my rhythm by

____.

Clinician threshold (fill in):

If I sleep less than _____ hours for _____ nights, I will treat it as yellow zone and contact my psychiatrist/therapist. (American Psychiatric Association, 2022; Harvey, 2008)

Chapter 8
When Your Tools Aren't Enough — Planning for Escalation

Anchor 8: Contingency - I plan for escalation with dignity.

Most people want to believe they will always be able to pull themselves back.

They want to believe that if they try hard enough—if they use their coping skills, their routines, their prayer, their journaling, their exercise—they will always be able to stop a spiral.

Sometimes that is true.
Sometimes your tools are enough.

And sometimes they are not.

This chapter is for the moments when your usual tools do not work quickly enough, when insight narrows, when your nervous system is driving, and the cost is rising.

Planning for escalation is not pessimism.
It is maturity.

It is your stable self protecting your vulnerable self.

Evidence-informed guidelines emphasize long-term planning, monitoring, and clear steps for escalation when needed. ^(Frank et al., 2005; Miklowitz et al., 2007)

This chapter helps you build those steps with dignity.

The uncomfortable truth: you can lose decision-making power in crisis

When symptoms escalate—especially in severe mania, mixed states, or severe depression—your ability to evaluate risk, tolerate boundaries, and accept help can change. ^(Miklowitz, 2008)

This can feel humiliating to admit.
It can also save your life.

If you have ever looked back after an episode and thought:
"I can't believe I did that,"
or
"Why didn't I get help sooner?"
you already know what this chapter is about.

You are not weak for needing a plan.
You are wise for making one while you are well.

Why crisis planning protects autonomy

Here is something many people do not realize until they have lived it:

If you do not make a plan while stable, the system makes one for you when you are unstable.

And the system is often not gentle.

When you arrive in an emergency setting in crisis,
you can lose control over:
- where you go
- who you talk to
- what information is shared
- what happens next
- how long decisions take

That is not always because providers are unkind.
It is because emergency systems are built for safety,
not personal preference.

So if you want more autonomy, you plan earlier.

A good contingency plan does not guarantee you will
never be hospitalized.
But it does increase the odds that if higher care is
needed, the path will be clearer, calmer, and less
traumatic. (Frank et al., 2005; Miklowitz et al., 2007)

The goal is not to avoid help; the goal is to avoid chaos

Some readers hear "contingency plan" and think it
means:
"I'm preparing to fail."

Not at all.

A contingency plan says:
"I'm preparing to stay safe."

The goal is to reduce:
- delay
- confusion
- panic
- argument
- relationship rupture
- emergency improvisation (Frank et al., 2005; Miklowitz et al., 2007)

The goal is to protect:
- safety
- dignity
- relationships
- finances and responsibilities
- your future

The three zones of escalation (simple and useful)

Most people need a three-level plan:

Green Zone (stable)
You are sleeping, functioning, and thinking clearly enough to make wise decisions.
You build the plan here.

Yellow Zone (early warning)
You are noticing warning signs, but you still have enough insight to respond.
This is where you have the most leverage. (Harvey, 2008)

Red Zone (tools aren't enough)
Insight narrows, symptoms escalate, risk rises.

This is where the plan becomes a lifeline. (Frank et al., 2005; Miklowitz et al., 2007)

What a real contingency plan includes

A meaningful plan is not just:
"Call me if I'm manic."

A meaningful plan answers practical questions:

1) What are my early warning signs (yellow zone)? (Harvey, 2008)

2) What are my red zone signs (escalation markers)? (Miklowitz, 2008; Frank et al., 2005; Miklowitz et al., 2007)

3) What steps do I take first in yellow zone? (Frank et al., 2005; Miklowitz et al., 2007; American Psychiatric Association, 2022)

4) When do I contact my psychiatrist/therapist? (thresholds) (Frank et al., 2005; Miklowitz et al., 2007; Harvey, 2008)

5) Who are my support people, and what are their roles? (National Institute for Health and Care Excellence, 2014; Frank, 2007)

6) What guardrails activate (spending, driving, social media, decisions)? (Frank et al., 2005; Miklowitz et al., 2007)

7) If urgent evaluation is needed, where do I go? (Frank et al., 2005; Miklowitz et al., 2007)

8) If hospitalization is needed, what is my preferred plan? (Frank et al., 2005; Miklowitz et al., 2007)

9) How do I protect responsibilities (kids, pets, work, bills)?

10) What does recovery and repair look like after? (National Institute for Health and Care Excellence, 2014; Frank, 2007)

Hospital planning: talking about it while stable

Many people avoid the topic of hospitalization
because it feels terrifying or shameful.
But avoiding the topic does not eliminate the
possibility.
It only removes your voice from the process.

If you and your treatment team agree that
hospitalization might be needed in certain red zone
scenarios, it can be wise to plan:
- what facilities you prefer (if you have options)
- what your psychiatrist recommends as the best
pathway (direct admission vs. ER vs. crisis clinic)
- who advocates for you if you are overwhelmed
- what medications and history should be
communicated
- what discharge planning should include (follow-up
appointments, sleep protection, support schedule)
(Frank et al., 2005; Miklowitz et al., 2007)

This planning can reduce trauma and increase
dignity.

"But what if my family uses this against me?"

This is a real fear for some people—especially if
family relationships are controlling or shaming.

A contingency plan does not require you to give every person access to every detail.

You decide:
- who is in your inner circle
- what permissions you give
- what information can be shared
- what steps you want others to take (National Institute for Health and Care Excellence, 2014; Frank, 2007)

If your family is unsafe, build your inner circle with clinicians, trusted friends, and chosen supports.

Your plan belongs to you.

The most important phrase in this chapter

Write it down if you need to:

"I will not wait until I'm in red zone to ask for help."
(Frank et al., 2005; Miklowitz et al., 2007; Harvey, 2008)

Waiting feels brave.
But often it is fear.

Early help is not weakness.
Early help is prevention.

How to introduce the plan to your support people

Support people panic when they do not know what to do.

They also panic when they feel responsible for everything.

A plan gives supporters a role—and boundaries.

You can say:
"I'm building a contingency plan while I'm stable. I'm not asking you to fix me. I'm asking you to follow a plan with me if I start to shift." (National Institute for Health and Care Excellence, 2014; Frank, 2007)

Then share only what they need:
- your yellow signs
- your red signs
- your first steps
- who to call and when

Where we are going next

In Chapter 9, we will talk about repair without shame—how to take responsibility for impact, rebuild trust, and protect relationships without drowning in self-hatred. (National Institute for Health and Care Excellence, 2014; Frank, 2007)

Anchor Check — Chapter 8 [Frank, 2007]

"When I am stable, I am willing to build or update my contingency plan with my therapist/support team so my vulnerable self is protected." [Frank et al., 2005; Miklowitz et al., 2007]

Go to Appendix A to create your contingency plan.

Chapter 9
Repair Without Shame —
Relationships, Accountability, and
Boundaries

Anchor 9: Repair - I repair without shame and rebuild trust over time.

If bipolar disorder has touched your relationships, you are not alone.

Many people living with bipolar disorder carry a specific kind of grief:
The grief of looking back and seeing damage they did not intend.
The grief of knowing they scared people they love.
The grief of realizing that even when you are trying your best, symptoms can still create fallout.

And then, layered on top of grief, shame often arrives.

Shame says:
"You don't deserve relationships."
"You're too much."
"You always ruin it."
"You should hide."

But shame does not repair anything.
Shame isolates.

Shame destroys motivation.
Shame makes it harder to tell the truth.

This chapter is about a different path:
repair without shame.

You can take responsibility for impact without
turning yourself into a monster.
You can rebuild trust without self-hatred.
You can create boundaries that protect both stability
and love. ^(National Institute for Health and Care Excellence, 2014; Frank, 2007)

Accountability and shame are not the same

Accountability says:
"I did that. It impacted you. I want to make it right."

Shame says:
"I am bad. I am unsafe. I should disappear."

Accountability leads to change.
Shame usually leads to hiding.

This distinction matters because bipolar disorder
often creates a painful dynamic:
people want to apologize, but the apology turns into
self-condemnation.
The other person is left holding both the original hurt
and the responsibility of comforting the apologizer.

That is not repair.
That is reversal.

Repair is not asking people to rescue you from your guilt.
Repair is taking ownership and building a different pattern.

A truth about trust: it rebuilds slower than symptoms improve

Sometimes people with bipolar disorder stabilize medically, and then feel frustrated that relationships are still tense.

You might think:
"I'm better now. Why aren't you over it?"

But trust does not rebuild at the same speed as mood. Trust rebuilds through consistent experiences over time. (National Institute for Health and Care Excellence, 2014; Frank, 2007)

Family-focused work emphasizes communication skills, relapse planning, and structured support because trust is strengthened by predictability, not promises. (National Institute for Health and Care Excellence, 2014; Frank, 2007)

A hard truth and a hopeful truth:
- Hard: you may not be able to repair everything quickly.
- Hopeful: you can repair more than you think through consistent stability practices.

The repair cycle: what to do after an episode

After an episode, many people either:
1) avoid the topic completely (because it hurts), or
2) try to fix everything at once (and overwhelm everyone).

Repair becomes more effective when you follow a steady sequence.

Step 1: Stabilize first
If you are still in yellow or red zone, do not start deep repair conversations.
Protect sleep and regulation first. (American Psychiatric Association, 2022)

A simple boundary:
"We will talk about this when we are both regulated."

That is not avoidance.
That is wise timing.

Step 2: Name what happened (without argument)
This is not the moment to debate memories.
This is the moment to acknowledge impact.

"I know I scared you when I ___________."
"I know I hurt you when I ___________."

Short. Clear. No defense.

Step 3: Validate the impact
Validation is not agreeing with every interpretation.
Validation is acknowledging that their experience
makes sense.

"It makes sense that you felt unsafe."
"It makes sense that you didn't know what to do."
"It makes sense that you're cautious now."

Step 4: Own your part (without self-hatred)
Ownership sounds like:
"I am responsible for that choice."
"I am responsible for how I spoke to you."
"I am responsible for getting help earlier."

Ownership does not require you to say:
"I am worthless."

Step 5: Offer a specific change (not a vague
promise)
Vague promises sound like:
"I'll never do that again."
"I'll try harder."

Specific changes sound like:
"When my sleep drops below _____ hours for _____
nights, I will contact my psychiatrist." (Frank et al., 2005;
Miklowitz et al., 2007; Harvey, 2008)

"I will not have major conversations after wind-down
starts." (American Psychiatric Association, 2022)
"I will activate our contingency plan earlier." (Frank et al.,

2005; Miklowitz et al., 2007)

"I will hand over my credit card during red zone if we agreed to that in advance." (Frank et al., 2005; Miklowitz et al., 2007)

Specificity builds trust.

Step 6: Ask what they need (and listen)
This is the part people often skip.

"What would help you feel safer in the future?"
"What would you want me to do sooner next time?"
"What boundaries do you need?" (National Institute for Health and Care Excellence, 2014; Frank, 2007)

Listening does not mean you agree to everything. It means you gather information about what trust requires.

Repair scripts you can actually use

Here are a few sentences you can borrow.

Script A: Truth + impact + change
"I'm sorry for __________. I understand it impacted you by __________. Here is what I'm changing: __________." (National Institute for Health and Care Excellence, 2014; Frank, 2007)

Script B: Naming the plan
"I'm not asking you to trust me because I said 'sorry.' I'm asking you to watch me follow a plan. I want stability to be something you can see." (Frank et al., 2005;

Miklowitz et al., 2007; National Institute for Health and Care Excellence, 2014; Frank, 2007)

Script C: If they're still angry
"You have a right to be angry. I'm not going to argue with your pain. I'm going to keep doing the work and keep showing up." (National Institute for Health and Care Excellence, 2014; Frank, 2007)

Boundaries that protect both stability and relationships

Sometimes people hear "boundaries" and think it means:
"I'm cutting everyone off."

But boundaries can also mean:
"I want us to stay connected without destroying each other."

Examples of protective boundaries:
- No yelling, name-calling, or threats.
- No major decisions at night. (American Psychiatric Association, 2022)

- No arguing during yellow/red zone; return later.
- If a conversation escalates, we pause for _____ minutes.
- If I'm not sleeping, we prioritize calm and clinical

contact instead of fighting. <sup>(Frank et al., 2005; Miklowitz et al., 2007;
American Psychiatric Association, 2022; Harvey, 2008)</sup>

Boundaries are especially important because conflict can be a trigger.
Boundaries reduce trigger stacking.

When repair is not possible (and what to do then)

Not every relationship will repair.
Some people are not safe.
Some relationships are abusive, exploitative, or controlling.
Some people will use your diagnosis as a weapon.

In those cases, repair does not mean staying.
Repair may mean leaving with clarity and support.

If you are unsure, discuss it with your therapist.
Your safety matters. ^(Frank et al., 2005; Miklowitz et al., 2007)

A gentle final truth: you can become trustworthy again

If you have done harm, it is normal to fear you are permanently disqualified from love.

But people rebuild trust every day.
Not through perfection.
Through honesty, humility, consistency, and follow-through.

Bipolar disorder may create storms.
But storms do not have to erase your identity or your future.

You can be a person who repairs.
You can be a person who learns.
You can be a person who follows a plan.

Where we are going next

In Chapter 10, we focus on decision-making guardrails—practical boundaries that protect your life when your brain state is vulnerable, especially around money, relationships, and major choices. (Frank et al., 2005; Miklowitz et al., 2007; American Psychiatric Association, 2022)

Anchor Check — Chapter 9 (Perry et al., 1999)

Write one repair sentence you could use (even if you never send it).

Truth + impact + change:
"I'm sorry for ___________________. I understand

it impacted you by ___________________. Here is

what I'm changing: _______________________."
(National Institute for Health and Care Excellence, 2014; Frank, 2007)

Circle one boundary you want to strengthen:
- no major conversations at night (American Psychiatric Association, 2022)

- pause when escalated
- follow the contingency plan earlier (Frank et al., 2005; Miklowitz et al., 2007)

- contact clinicians at thresholds (Frank et al., 2005; Miklowitz et al., 2007; Harvey, 2008)

- spending guardrails (Frank et al., 2005; Miklowitz et al., 2007)

Optional:
Who is one person you need to repair with slowly, over time (not in one conversation)?

____

____

Chapter 10
Decision-Making During Vulnerable Seasons — Guardrails That Protect Your Life

Anchor 10: Guardrails - I do not make permanent decisions inside temporary states.

Anchor 10: Do not make permanent decisions inside temporary states.

Bipolar disorder does not only affect mood.
It can affect decision-making.

When your brain state shifts, your perception of risk can shift.
Your tolerance for consequences can shift.
Your sense of urgency can shift.
What feels "obviously right" can be profoundly different from what your stable self would choose.
(Miklowitz, 2008; Frank et al., 2005; Miklowitz et al., 2007)

That is why you need guardrails.

Guardrails are not a lack of freedom.
Guardrails are how you protect freedom.

This chapter will help you build decision rules that keep your life from being remade by a temporary state.

Why guardrails are an act of dignity

Some people resist guardrails because they feel like:
- control
- punishment
- evidence that they cannot be trusted
- a loss of spontaneity

But the truth is: wise people build guardrails.

People build guardrails for:
- addiction recovery
- chronic health conditions
- financial stability
- parenting safety
- leadership integrity

Guardrails do not mean you are broken.
Guardrails mean you are planning for reality.

Evidence-informed guidelines emphasize planning, monitoring, and risk management as part of bipolar disorder care. (Frank et al., 2005; Miklowitz et al., 2007)
Guardrails are one practical form of that planning.

The "state-based decision" problem

Here is the pattern many people with bipolar disorder recognize:

When you are up-shifted, you may:
- feel unusually confident

- feel destined for something
- feel impatient with limits
- feel compelled to act now
- take risks that feel "worth it"
- believe you do not need input [Miklowitz, 2008]

When you are down-shifted, you may:
- feel hopeless
- feel like nothing matters
- believe your future is already ruined
- feel like leaving or quitting is the only relief [Miklowitz, 2008]

When you are mixed or agitated, you may:
- feel urgency + despair
- feel trapped and reactive
- make impulsive decisions just to escape the feeling [Miklowitz, 2008]

In each case, the danger is the same:
making permanent decisions inside temporary states.

So we adopt a rule:
"I will not make identity decisions inside a state."

Guardrails are "pre-decisions" made while well

A guardrail is a decision you make while stable so you do not have to negotiate with your symptoms later.

It sounds like:
- "If I'm not sleeping, I don't make big decisions."

110

(American Psychiatric Association, 2022)

- "If I'm in a yellow zone, I delay major purchases." (Frank et al., 2005; Miklowitz et al., 2007)

- "If I'm in red zone, my support person holds my cards." (Frank et al., 2005; Miklowitz et al., 2007)

- "If I'm feeling hopeless, I don't quit my job that week." (Frank et al., 2005; Miklowitz et al., 2007)

Guardrails are the stable self speaking for the vulnerable self.

The five high-risk decision categories

If you only put guardrails around five areas, put them around these:

1) Money
2) Relationships
3) Work and school
4) Travel and mobility
5) Public presence (social media, reputation)

These are the areas where an episode can create long-lasting consequences.

Money guardrails (practical and non-shaming)

Many people with bipolar disorder experience impulsive spending during hypomania/mania.
Not always because they are reckless, but because risk perception and reward seeking can shift. (Miklowitz, 2008; Frank et al., 2005; Miklowitz et al., 2007)

Money guardrails are not about shame.
They are about protecting your future self from debt, legal issues, and regret.

Examples of money guardrails:
- No purchases over $____ without a 24–72 hour waiting period. (Frank et al., 2005; Miklowitz et al., 2007)
- No new credit cards or loans during yellow/red zone. (Frank et al., 2005; Miklowitz et al., 2007)
- No online shopping after wind-down time. (American Psychiatric Association, 2022)
- Spending alerts on accounts.
- A trusted person receives a notification if spending rises beyond a limit (only if you consent).
- Cards temporarily held by support person during red zone (if agreed in advance). (Frank et al., 2005; Miklowitz et al., 2007)

The goal is not to eliminate generosity or joy.
The goal is to make sure generosity does not become self-destruction.

Relationship guardrails (especially in intensity)

Episodes can intensify emotions and certainty.
You may feel like:
- "This relationship is everything."
or
- "This relationship is over."

Guardrail:
No breakups, divorces, major romantic decisions, or relational ultimatums in yellow/red zone.
Talk to your therapist first. (Frank et al., 2005; Miklowitz et al., 2007; National Institute for Health and Care Excellence, 2014; Frank, 2007)

Another guardrail:
No major relationship conversations after wind-down starts. (American Psychiatric Association, 2022)

This is not avoidance.
This is choosing timing that protects both people.

Work and calling guardrails (purpose without whiplash)

Work decisions are often tied to identity.
That makes them vulnerable during mood shifts.

Guardrails might include:
- No quitting a job without a 7-day wait period + therapist conversation. (Frank et al., 2005; Miklowitz et al., 2007)
- No taking on new major commitments if sleep is disrupted. (American Psychiatric Association, 2022)
- No launching a major project alone; review with support person first.
- In depression, commit to "minimum viable functioning" rather than scorched-earth resignation.

Guardrails protect your calling from your chemistry.

Travel and mobility guardrails

Travel can disrupt rhythm and sleep—two stabilizers for many people with bipolar disorder. (American Psychiatric Association, 2022; Miklowitz et al., 2007; Rea et al., 2003)

Guardrails might include:
- No last-minute travel when sleep is unstable.
- Maintain wake time as much as possible.
- Plan time zone shifts intentionally.
- Check in with clinician before major travel if you have history of travel-triggered episodes. (Frank et al., 2005; Miklowitz et al., 2007)

Again: not restriction—protection.

Public presence guardrails (social media, visibility, reputation)

In up-shift states, people often post more, share more, argue more, or make big announcements.
In down-shift states, people may post despair, hopelessness, or impulsive confessions.

Guardrails might include:
- No major social media posts after 9 p.m.
- No public announcements in yellow/red zone.
- One trusted person reviews major posts if you want that support.
- If you are in red zone, you log out and hand the

password to a trusted person temporarily (only if safe and agreed). (Frank et al., 2005; Miklowitz et al., 2007)

Your future self deserves protection from your temporary state self.

A clinician-supported guardrail: "If I'm not sleeping, I treat it like data"

Sleep disruption is often a warning sign and destabilizer. (American Psychiatric Association, 2022; Miklowitz et al., 2007)
So a powerful guardrail is:
If I'm not sleeping, I do not argue with my brain.
I treat it as clinical data and act early.

That action might include:
- reducing stimulation
- tightening rhythm
- contacting my psychiatrist/therapist at thresholds
(Frank et al., 2005; Miklowitz et al., 2007; Harvey, 2008)

How to build guardrails without losing your sense of self

Guardrails should be:
- simple
- specific
- written down
- shared with inner circle
- adjusted over time

They should not be 50 rules you resent.
They should be 5–10 protections you respect.

A good test:
Do these guardrails protect my values and my future?

If yes, they are not punishment.
They are wisdom.

Where we are going next

In Chapter 11, we return to meaning and purpose: how to build a life that fits your brain, how to pursue goals without destabilizing, and how to define "normal" in a way that is honest and hopeful. (Miklowitz et al., 2007; Rea et al., 2003)

Anchor Check — Chapter 10 (McCarthy et al., 2021)

Choose ONE guardrail to put in writing today.

My guardrail:

"If _________________________________ (warning sign),

then I will ___________________________________
(protective action)." (Frank et al., 2005; Miklowitz et al., 2007; American
Psychiatric Association, 2022)

Examples:

- If I sleep less than ___ hours for ___ nights, then I
will delay big decisions and contact my psychiatrist.
(American Psychiatric Association, 2022; Harvey, 2008)

- If I feel urgent and grand, then I will wait 72 hours
before spending over $____. (Frank et al., 2005; Miklowitz et al., 2007)
- If I feel hopeless, then I will call my therapist before
making major life changes. (Frank et al., 2005; Miklowitz et al., 2007)

One support person who can help me keep this
guardrail is:

_______________ ___________________________.

(National Institute for Health and Care Excellence, 2014; Frank, 2007)

Chapter 11
Meaning, Purpose, and a Life Bigger Than the Diagnosis

Anchor 11: Meaning - I build a life bigger than the diagnosis.

Anchor 11: Build a life bigger than the diagnosis.

If you have made it this far, you have probably felt two competing fears at different times:

Fear #1: "This diagnosis will take everything from me."
Fear #2: "If I take stability seriously, my life will become small."

Both fears make sense.

Bipolar disorder can be costly.
And stability can feel, at first, like limitation.

But the aim of anchored living is not to shrink your life.
The aim is to build a life that fits your brain—so you can keep what matters and grow what is good.

This chapter is about meaning, purpose, and identity: how to pursue a meaningful life without destabilizing, and how to hold your diagnosis without letting it swallow you.

A stable life is not a boring life

Some people equate stability with blandness.

They miss:
- intensity
- spontaneity
- the rush of big plans
- the feeling of being "on fire"

If you have ever missed an up-shift state, you are not alone.
That grief deserves honesty.

But stability is not the absence of passion.
Stability is passion that does not destroy your relationships, finances, health, and future. (Frank et al., 2005; Miklowitz et al., 2007)

There is a difference between:
- a life that is alive, and
- a life that is chaotic.

Anchors protect aliveness.

The difference between "normal" and "healthy for you"

Many people living with bipolar disorder secretly measure themselves against a standard that was never built for their nervous system:
- irregular sleep

- constant hustle
- social intensity every night
- frequent travel
- caffeine all day
- emotional whiplash in relationships
- decisions made quickly, publicly, and impulsively

That standard is not "normal."
It is modern chaos.

A healthier question is:
"What is healthy for my brain?" (Miklowitz et al., 2007; Rea et al., 2003)

This is where rhythm-based approaches are so helpful.
They teach you to build daily structure that supports long-term mood stability, without turning you into a robot. (Miklowitz et al., 2007; Rea et al., 2003)

Purpose without pressure: building a life that doesn't trigger episodes

A meaningful life involves challenge.
But some kinds of challenge are destabilizing.

The goal is not to avoid all stress.
The goal is to avoid stress that consistently triggers shifts.

This is where your episode signature (Chapter 5) becomes a gift.

You learn which patterns tend to push you:
- too many commitments
- too little sleep
- overstimulation
- conflict spirals
- seasons of grief and transition
- long periods without rest (Frank et al., 2005; Miklowitz et al., 2007; American Psychiatric Association, 2022)

Then you build purpose with protection.

A simple rule:
If pursuing a goal regularly costs you sleep and rhythm, you need a different strategy—not more determination. (American Psychiatric Association, 2022; Miklowitz et al., 2007)

Your values: the core of identity that outlasts a state

One of the most stabilizing identity practices is values-based living:
a commitment to the kind of person you want to be, regardless of mood state.

Values might include:
- honesty
- faithfulness
- compassion
- courage
- stability
- humility
- service

- creativity
- stewardship
- connection

Values are different from feelings.
Feelings shift.
Values guide.

In vulnerable states, you may not feel like your values
are accessible.
That is why you write them down and build supports
around them.

A practical values exercise (quick and powerful)

Choose 3 values that you want your life to be
anchored to:

1) ____

2) ____

3) ____

Now ask:
"What does this value look like when I am stable?"
"What does it look like when I am vulnerable?"
"What supports help me live it?"

For example:
If your value is "stewardship," a support might be a

money guardrail. (Frank et al., 2005; Miklowitz et al., 2007)

If your value is "faithfulness," a support might be the "no major conversations at night" rule. (American Psychiatric Association, 2022)

If your value is "compassion," a support might be early help-seeking so your loved ones don't carry unnecessary cost. (Frank et al., 2005; Miklowitz et al., 2007; Harvey, 2008)

Values turn anchors into meaning.

The role of community in meaning

A meaningful life usually involves connection.
Even if you are introverted.
Even if you have been hurt.
Even if you fear being a burden.

Family-focused and psychoeducation approaches repeatedly highlight the value of informed support and stable relationship patterns in improving outcomes. (National Institute for Health and Care Excellence, 2014; Frank, 2007; Perry et al., 1999)

Meaning is harder in isolation.
Not because you are weak.
Because humans are built for connection.

When faith is part of meaning (and when it isn't)

If faith is part of your life, it can be a powerful meaning anchor.
It can also be misused against you.

Healthy faith support:
- honors psychiatry and therapy as part of wisdom
- supports rhythms that protect stability
- avoids shame and spiritual threats
- offers compassion and accountability

If faith is not part of your life, you can still build
meaning through:
- relationships
- service
- creative work
- purpose-driven goals
- community involvement
- personal integrity

Meaning is not owned by one worldview.
Meaning is built by living aligned with what matters
to you.

A vision for your future (realistic and hopeful)

You may not get to choose whether you have bipolar
disorder.
But you can choose:
- whether you build a team
- whether you protect rhythm
- whether you respond early
- whether you plan for escalation
- whether you repair after storms

- whether you build guardrails that protect your future ^(Frank et al., 2005; Miklowitz et al., 2007)

Those choices add up.

A future with bipolar disorder can include:
- stable relationships
- meaningful work
- integrity
- joy
- connection
- rest
- growth
- purpose

Not because the illness disappears.
Because you become anchored.

Where we are going next

In Chapter 12, we pull the entire book together into a stability plan you can review regularly: a chapter-map summary, a personal anchor checklist, and a practical "what to do next" pathway for ongoing maintenance.

(Frank et al., 2005; Miklowitz et al., 2007)

Anchor Check — Chapter 11 ^(Rea et al., 2003)

Write your "life bigger than the diagnosis" sentence (one line):

"My life is bigger than bipolar disorder because I am committed to ______________________________."

Choose 3 values you want to anchor to:

1) ____

2) ____

3) ____

One way I will protect purpose without destabilizing is:

____

____

Optional:
Who helps you remember who you are when symptoms try to rewrite your story?

____

____

Chapter 12
Your Ongoing Stability Plan — Putting the Anchors Together

Anchor 12: Ongoing plan - I revisit and refine my stability plan.

Anchor 12: Revisit and refine your stability plan.

This chapter is a landing place.

You have learned a lot so far:
- how to separate identity from diagnosis
- how to treat bipolar disorder as a brain health condition
- how to build a care team
- how to build a support circle
- how to map your episode signature
- how to identify warning signs and respond early
- how to protect sleep and rhythm
- how to plan for escalation
- how to repair without shame
- how to build guardrails that protect your future
- how to hold meaning and purpose without destabilizing

Now we pull it together into a stability plan you can revisit—especially when life becomes noisy.

Because the goal is not to read this book once and feel inspired.
The goal is to build a plan you can use for years.

Guidelines emphasize long-term management, monitoring, and relapse prevention planning in bipolar disorder. (Frank et al., 2005; Miklowitz et al., 2007)
This chapter is your practical framework for that reality.

A reminder: stability is built in ordinary days

Most people imagine stability is built in crisis.
But crisis is where you spend stability.

Stability is built in ordinary days:
- showing up to appointments
- taking medication consistently (as prescribed)
- protecting sleep and rhythm
- lowering trigger stacking
- staying connected to support
- repairing quickly when conflict starts
- using guardrails to prevent expensive decisions (Frank et al., 2005; Miklowitz et al., 2007; American Psychiatric Association, 2022; Miklowitz et al., 2007; Rea et al., 2003)

It is not dramatic. It is faithful.

1) The anchor I most need to strengthen right now is (circle one):

Identity / Understanding / Team / Support / Signature / Early response / Rhythm / Contingency / Repair / Guardrails / Meaning / Ongoing plan

2) My next step (one sentence):
This week, I will

____

3) One person who will know my plan is:

____

Appendix A
Contingency Plan Worksheet

1) What are my early warning signs (yellow zone)?

2) What are my red zone signs (escalation markers)?

3) What steps do I take first in yellow zone?

4) When do I contact my psychiatrist/therapist?

5) Who are my support people, and what are their roles?

6) What guardrails activate (spending, driving, social media, decisions)?

7) If urgent evaluation is needed, where do I go?

8) If hospitalization is needed, what is my preferred plan?

9) How do I protect responsibilities (kids, pets, work, bills)?

10) What does recovery and repair look like after?

Appendix B:
All Anchors at a Glance

Anchor 1: Identity - You are not your diagnosis.

Anchor 2: Understanding - This is a brain health condition with patterns.

Anchor 3: Team - I do not manage this alone.

Anchor 4: Support - I build a wise circle and healthy boundaries.

Anchor 5: Signature - I know my pattern.

Anchor 6: Early response - I catch shifts early and act sooner.

Anchor 7: Rhythm - I protect sleep and daily rhythms.

Anchor 8: Contingency - I plan for escalation with dignity.

Anchor 9: Repair - I repair without shame and rebuild trust over time.

Anchor 10: Guardrails - I do not make permanent decisions inside temporary states.

Anchor 11: Meaning - I build a life bigger than the diagnosis.

Anchor 12: Ongoing plan - I revisit and refine my stability plan.

References

American Psychiatric Association. (2022). Diagnostic and statistical manual of mental disorders (5th ed., text rev.; DSM-5-TR). Author.

Colom, F., Vieta, E., Martínez-Arán, A., Reinares, M., Goikolea, J. M., Benabarre, A., & Corominas, J. (2003). A randomized trial on the efficacy of group psychoeducation in the prophylaxis of recurrences in bipolar patients whose disease is in remission. Archives of General Psychiatry, 60(4), 402–407.

Frank, E., Kupfer, D. J., Thase, M. E., Mallinger, A. G., Swartz, H. A., Fagiolini, A. M., Grochocinski, V. J., Houck, P., Scott, J., Thompson, W., & Monk, T. (2005). Two-year outcomes for interpersonal and social rhythm therapy in individuals with bipolar I disorder. Archives of General Psychiatry, 62(9), 996–1004.

Frank, E. (2007). Interpersonal and social rhythm therapy: An intervention addressing rhythm dysregulation in bipolar disorder. Dialogues in Clinical Neuroscience, 9(3), 325–332.

Harvey, A. G. (2008). Sleep disturbance in bipolar disorder: Therapeutic implications. American Journal of Psychiatry, 165(7), 830–843.

McCarthy, M. J., Gottlieb, J. F., Gonzalez, R., et al. (2021). Neurobiological and behavioral mechanisms of circadian rhythm disruption in bipolar disorder: A critical multidisciplinary literature review and agenda for future research from the ISBD task force on chronobiology. Bipolar Disorders.

Miklowitz, D. J., Otto, M. W., Frank, E., Reilly-Harrington, N. A., Kogan, J. N., Sachs, G. S., & STEP-BD Investigators. (2007). Intensive psychosocial intervention enhances functioning in patients with bipolar depression: Results from a 9-month randomized controlled trial. American Journal of Psychiatry, 164(9), 1340–1347.

Miklowitz, D. J., Otto, M. W., Frank, E., Reilly-Harrington, N. A., Wisniewski, S. R., Kogan, J. N., Nierenberg, A. A., Calabrese, J. R., Marangell, L. B., Gyulai, L., Araga, M., Gonzalez, J. M., Shirley, E. R., Thase, M. E., & Sachs, G. S. (2007). Psychosocial treatments for bipolar depression: A 1-year randomized trial from the Systematic Treatment Enhancement Program. Archives of General Psychiatry, 64(4), 419–426.

Miklowitz, D. J. (2008). Bipolar disorder: A family-focused treatment approach (2nd ed.). Guilford Press.

National Institute for Health and Care Excellence. (2014). Bipolar disorder: Assessment and management (NICE Guideline CG 85). National Institute for Health and Care Excellence.

Perry, A., Tarrier, N., Morriss, R., McCarthy, E., & Limb, K. (1999). Randomised controlled trial of efficacy of teaching patients with bipolar disorder to identify early symptoms of relapse and obtain treatment. BMJ, 318, 149–153.

Rea, M. M., Tompson, M. C., Miklowitz, D. J., Goldstein, M. J., Hwang, S., & Mintz, J. (2003). Family-focused treatment versus individual treatment for bipolar disorder: Results of a randomized clinical trial. Journal of Consulting and Clinical Psychology, 71(3), 482–492.

Yatham, L. N., Kennedy, S. H., Parikh, S. V., Schaffer, A., Bond, D. J., Frey, B. N., … Ravindran, A. V. (2018). Canadian Network for Mood and Anxiety Treatments (CANMAT) and International Society for Bipolar Disorders (ISBD) 2018 guidelines for the management of patients with bipolar disorder. Bipolar Disorders, 20(2), 97–170.

About the Author

Cindy H. Carr, D.Min., MACL, has spent her vocational life walking alongside people in the slow, often unseen work of formation and change. Her career has been intentionally bi-vocational, shaped by years of pastoring, business leadership, and pastoral counseling—always with a focus on helping people live with greater clarity, dignity, and wholeness.

She earned a Master of Arts in Church Leadership from Eastern Mennonite Seminary and completed her doctoral work at Liberty University. Over the years, she served multiple churches in Virginia's Shenandoah Valley in a variety of pastoral and leadership capacities.

In this season of life, Cindy's work has shifted from direct leadership into writing and education. Through her books, she helps readers implement formation-based principles she has taught throughout her career—practices centered on identity, connection, return, and steady growth without shame.

Learn more about Cindy and her work at
CindyHCarr.com